FROM DIAGNOSIS TO RECOVERY

Overcoming Cancer and Finding Renewed Purpose

Copyright © [2023] [Leonard Irving]

COPYRIGHT PAGE

This work is owned by [Angelo Press] and is protected by copyright laws. Without the written consent of the copyright holder, it cannot be duplicated, copied, or disseminated in any way. This work's unauthorized use or dissemination is punishable by both civil and criminal laws.

TABLE OF CONTENTS

UNDERSTANDING CANCER
- INTRODUCTION
- WHAT IS CANCER
- COMMON TYPES OF CANCER
- CANCER STAGES AND DETECTION METHODS
- CAUSES AND RISK FACTORS OF CANCER

THE EMOTIONAL JOURNEY OF DEALING WITH CANCER
- COPING WITH THE SHOCK OF CANCER DIAGNOSIS
- FINDING HOPE AND PURPOSE THROUGH CANCER
- SEEKING MEDICAL TREATMENT AND SUPPORT

THE PHYSICAL JOURNEY OF DEALING WITH CANCER
- CANCER TREATMENT OPTIONS
- COPING WITH THE SIDE EFFECTS OF CANCER TREATMENT
- COPING WITH EMOTIONAL AND MENTAL HEALTH CHANGES

LIFESTYLE CHANGES
- A HOLISTIC APPROACH TO RECOVERY
- NUTRITION AND CANCER: EATING FOR HEALTH

- EXERCISE AND CANCER: MOVING TOWARD WELLNESS
- SLEEP, STRESS, AND OTHER LIFESTYLE FACTORS
- PROVIDING SELF-CARE DURING RECOVERY
- SUPPORT SYSTEMS

MOVING FORWARD
- FINDING MEANING AND PURPOSE
- FINDING HOPE AND INSPIRATION IN YOUR JOURNEY
- REFLECTING ON YOUR LIFE AND VALUES
- CELEBRATING MILESTONES AND ACCOMPLISHMENTS
- MANAGING FEAR AND ANXIETY ABOUT RECURRENCE
- EMBRACING LIFE AFTER CANCER

CONCLUSION
- THE JOURNEY OF HEALING: A CONTINUING PROCESS
- APPENDIX: ADDITIONAL RESOURCES FOR CANCER PATIENTS AND CAREGIVERS

PART I

UNDERSTANDING CANCER

INTRODUCTION

Cancer is a word that strikes fear into the hearts of many people. It evokes images of sickness, pain, and death. It can strike anyone, at any age, regardless of their gender, ethnicity, or lifestyle choices. A cancer diagnosis can be overwhelming, and it can be difficult to know where to turn for information and support. But for those of us who have survived cancer, it represents something else entirely: hope, strength, and resilience. It is a badge of honor that we wear proudly, a testament to our ability to overcome adversity and come out on the other side stronger and more alive than ever before.

In this book, we will explore the journey of healing from cancer. We will discuss the physical, emotional, and spiritual aspects of cancer, and offer practical advice on how to navigate the challenges of cancer treatment and recovery.

In the pages that follow, you will meet people who have faced some of the most daunting odds imaginable. They have battled cancer while raising a family, running a business, or pursuing a dream. They have dealt with the physical and emotional toll of treatment, the fear of recurrence, and the uncertainty of the future. But through it all, they have discovered a strength they never knew they had, and a gratitude for life that they will never take for granted.

This book is also a tribute to the medical professionals who have dedicated their lives to fighting cancer. From oncologists to nurses to researchers, these heroes work tirelessly to find new treatments and cures. They offer hope and compassion to their patients, and inspire us all with their dedication to the fight against cancer.

Cancer can be a lonely and isolating experience, but it does not have to be. If you or someone you love has been touched by cancer, I hope that this book will provide comfort, support, and wisdom. Always remember that you are not alone in your struggle, and there is always hope for a better tomorrow. Together, we can overcome this disease and emerge stronger and more vibrant than ever before. So let these stories of survival and perseverance inspire you to keep fighting, to never give up, and to live each day to the fullest.

Finally, this book is a reminder that cancer can be beaten. It is not a death sentence, but a challenge. It is a journey that will test your strength and resilience, but in the end, it can also be a source of inspiration and hope.

WHAT IS CANCER

Cancer is a broad term used to describe the abnormal growth and division of cells within the body. Unlike normal cells that grow and divide in a controlled and orderly manner, cancer cells divide and grow uncontrollably, invading and damaging surrounding tissues and organs. These cells grow and divide uncontrollably, forming a mass of abnormal cells called a tumor.

Tumors can be benign or malignant. Benign tumors do not spread to other parts of the body, and once they are removed, they usually do not return. Malignant tumors, on the other hand, can invade nearby tissues and organs and can spread to other parts of the body through the bloodstream or lymphatic system.

Cancer can occur in any part of the body, and it can affect people of all ages, races, and genders. The causes of cancer are complex and can be influenced by many factors, including genetics, environmental factors, lifestyle choices, and exposure to certain chemicals and toxins.

COMMON TYPES OF CANCER

Cancer is a complex and multifaceted disease that affects millions of people worldwide. Understanding the common types of cancer and risk factors associated with the disease can help individuals take steps to prevent and detect cancer early, improving their chances of successful treatment and long-term survival.

There are over 100 different types of cancer, each characterized by a specific type of cell or tissue in which the cancer originates. Some of the most common types of cancer include:

BREAST CANCER

Breast cancer is the most common type of cancer among women worldwide, accounting for nearly one in four of all cancer cases. It occurs when cells in the breast tissue start to grow uncontrollably, forming a lump or mass, usually starting in the milk ducts or lobules.

There are several different types of breast cancer, including ductal carcinoma in situ (DCIS), invasive ductal carcinoma, and invasive lobular carcinoma. Risk factors for breast cancer include age, family history, certain genetic mutations, exposure to estrogen, and lifestyle factors such as obesity, alcohol consumption, and lack of physical activity.

Treatment options for breast cancer depend on the stage and type of cancer, but may include surgery, radiation therapy, chemotherapy, and hormone therapy.

LUNG CANCER

Lung cancer is the second most common type of cancer, and is responsible for the highest number of cancer-related deaths worldwide. The majority of lung cancers are caused by smoking, but exposure to secondhand smoke, air pollution, and radon gas can also increase the risk.

There are two main types of lung cancer: non-small cell lung cancer and small cell lung cancer. Symptoms of lung cancer include coughing, chest pain, shortness of breath, and coughing up blood.

Treatment options for lung cancer depend on the type and stage of cancer, but may include surgery, radiation therapy, chemotherapy, immunotherapy and targeted therapy.

COLORECTAL CANCER

Colorectal cancer is the third most common type of cancer in both men and women. It is a type of cancer that develops in the colon or rectum. Symptoms of colorectal cancer may include changes in bowel habits, abdominal pain, blood in the stool, and unexplained weight loss and risk factors for colorectal cancer include age, family history, a diet high in red or processed meat, smoking, and lack of physical activity.

Colorectal cancer can be prevented or detected early through regular screening tests, such as colonoscopies. Treatment options for colorectal cancer depend on the stage and type of cancer, but may include surgery, radiation therapy, chemotherapy, and targeted therapy.

PROSTATE CANCER

Prostate cancer is a type of cancer that develops in the prostate gland in men. It is the most common type of cancer among men, and typically develops in cells in the gland that produce semen.

Prostate cancer is typically slow-growing and may not cause symptoms for many years. Symptoms of prostate cancer may include difficulty urinating, blood in the urine or semen, and discomfort or pain in the pelvic area and risk factors for prostate cancer include age, family history, race, and lifestyle factors such as diet and exercise.

Treatment options for prostate cancer depend on the stage and type of cancer, but may include surgery, radiation therapy, chemotherapy, hormone therapy, and watchful waiting.

SKIN CANCER

Skin cancer is the most common type of cancer, with more than 3 million cases diagnosed each year in the United States. It typically develops in cells within the outer layer of skin, and is often caused by exposure to ultraviolet (UV) radiation from the sun or tanning beds.

There are several different types of skin cancer, including basal cell carcinoma, squamous cell carcinoma, and melanoma. Basal cell and squamous cell carcinomas are the most common and least dangerous types of skin cancer, while melanoma is a more aggressive form of skin cancer that can spread to other parts of the body if left untreated.

Risk factors for skin cancer include a history of sunburn, a large number of moles or freckles, a family history of skin cancer, and a weakened immune system. Prevention strategies include the use of sunscreen, protective clothing, and avoiding excessive exposure to the sun.

Other common types of cancer include pancreatic cancer, bladder cancer, kidney cancer, liver cancer, and ovarian cancer.

While the exact causes of cancer are not always known, certain risk factors can increase the likelihood of developing the disease. These include age, family history, exposure to certain chemicals or substances, obesity, and a weakened immune system.

Early detection and treatment are key to improving cancer outcomes. Regular screenings, such as mammograms, colonoscopies, and skin exams, can help detect cancer in its early stages when it is most treatable.

Treatment options for cancer depend on the type and stage of the disease, as well as the individual's overall health and preferences. Common treatments include surgery, radiation therapy, chemotherapy, targeted therapies, and immunotherapy.

In addition to medical treatment, many cancer patients find complementary and alternative therapies, such as acupuncture and meditation, helpful in managing symptoms and improving their quality of life.

CANCER STAGES AND DETECTION METHODS

Understanding cancer staging and detection is crucial for developing a treatment plan that is tailored to each individual's needs.

CANCER STAGING

Cancer staging is the process of determining how advanced a cancer is and how far it has spread in the body. Staging is an essential part of cancer diagnosis and treatment because it helps doctors understand the severity of the cancer and how best to treat it. The stage of cancer is determined by a combination of factors, including the size and location of the tumor, whether the cancer has spread to nearby tissue or lymph nodes, and whether it has spread to distant parts of the body. Once the cancer is staged, doctors can develop a treatment plan that is tailored to the individual's needs.

There are different staging systems for different types of cancer, but most use a similar system that involves five stages:

STAGE 0

Stage 0 is also known as carcinoma in situ (CIS). In this stage, cancer is limited to the tissue where it began, and it has not spread to nearby tissues. Most CIS forms of cancer have a high cure rate, and a complete removal of the abnormal tissue may be enough to prevent recurrence.

STAGE I
In stage I cancer, the tumor is usually small and localized, and it has not spread to nearby lymph nodes. Surgery is often the primary treatment for stage I cancer. Radiation therapy or chemotherapy may also be recommended.

STAGE II
In stage II cancer, the tumor has grown, and it may have invaded nearby tissues or organs. It may also have spread to nearby lymph nodes. A combination of treatments, such as surgery, radiation therapy, and chemotherapy, may be needed to treat stage II cancer.

STAGE III
In stage III cancer, the tumor is larger, and it has spread to nearby lymph nodes and other organs. Treatment options for stage III cancer may include surgery, radiation therapy, chemotherapy, or a combination of these treatments.

STAGE IV

Stage IV cancer is the most advanced stage of cancer. In this stage, cancer has spread beyond the primary site to other organs or tissues in the body. Treatment for stage IV cancer may include surgery, radiation therapy, chemotherapy, immunotherapy or a combination of these treatments.

DETECTION METHODS

Early detection is critical in treating cancer successfully. When cancer is detected at an early stage, it is more likely to be curable. There are several methods used to detect cancer in the body, including:

IMAGING TESTS

Imaging tests, such as X-rays, CT scans, MRI scans, and PET scans, are used to create images of the inside of the body. These tests can help doctors identify tumors and determine their location and size. Imaging tests are often used to screen for cancer and to monitor the progression of the disease.

Mammography is used to screen for breast cancer in women. It involves taking X-ray images of the breast tissue to identify any abnormalities or masses.

X-ray imaging is used to detect lung cancer by taking images of the chest to spot any abnormalities or masses.

CT scans generate detailed images of the body using X-rays to detect the presence of cancerous masses.

A PET scan is used to detect cancer by injecting a radioactive tracer into the bloodstream which is absorbed by the cancerous cells. The scan then picks up the radiation to create detailed images of the body.

BLOOD TESTS

Blood tests can help detect cancer markers, which are abnormal proteins produced by cancer cells. Blood tests are used to screen for certain types of cancer, such as prostate cancer and ovarian cancer. Examples of cancer marker tests include prostate-specific antigen (PSA) for prostate cancer, carcinoembryonic antigen (CEA) for colon cancer, and CA-125 for ovarian cancer. Abnormal levels of these substances can indicate the presence of cancer.

BIOPSY

A biopsy involves the removal of a small sample of tissue from the suspected cancerous area. The tissue is then examined under a microscope to determine whether it is cancerous. There are various biopsy methods available, including:

- **Needle biopsy** – a thin needle is inserted into the area to remove a small sample of tissue.

- **Endoscopic biopsy** – a thin, flexible tube with a camera and a tool for removing tissue is inserted through the mouth, rectum, or other small incisions to reach the suspected cancerous area.

- **Surgical biopsy** – a surgical procedure is used to remove the entire tumor or a portion of it.

GENETIC TESTING

Genetic testing can help detect inherited gene mutations that increase the risk of developing certain cancers, such as breast and ovarian cancer. It involves taking a sample of blood or tissue and analyzing it for mutations in specific genes that are associated with cancer. If a person tests positive for a cancer-associated gene mutation, they may be at an increased risk of developing cancer and may need to undergo more frequent screening.

ENDOSCOPY

Endoscopy is a procedure in which a thin, flexible tube with a camera attached is inserted into the body. The camera allows doctors to see inside the body and examine the digestive tract, lungs, or other organs for signs of cancer. Endoscopy is often used to diagnose cancers of the digestive tract, such as colon cancer.

PHYSICAL EXAMINATION

A physical examination is often the first step in diagnosing cancer. During a physical exam, a doctor will examine the body for lumps, bumps, or other signs of cancer. They may also check for enlarged lymph nodes, which can be a sign that cancer has spread to nearby tissue.

CAUSES AND RISK FACTORS OF CANCER

Here are some causes and risk factors of cancer, from environmental factors to inherited genetic mutations.

ENVIRONMENTAL FACTORS

Environmental factors play a significant role in the development of cancer. Exposure to certain chemicals, radiation, and pollution can damage DNA and lead to the formation of cancer cells. Some of the environmental factors that have been linked to cancer include:

- **Exposure To Tobacco Smoke**

Tobacco smoke contains over 70 carcinogens, including chemicals such as polycyclic aromatic hydrocarbons (PAHs) and nitrosamines. These chemicals can damage DNA and cause mutations that lead to cancer. Smoking is responsible for the majority of lung cancer cases, but it is also linked to many other types of cancer, including bladder, kidney, pancreas, and mouth cancer.

- **EXPOSURE TO UV RADIATION**

UV radiation from the sun or tanning beds can cause DNA damage and lead to the development of skin cancer. The most common types of skin cancer are basal cell carcinoma, squamous cell carcinoma, and melanoma.

- **EXPOSURE TO IONIZING RADIATION**

Ionizing radiation, such as X-rays and gamma rays, can damage DNA and cause mutations that lead to cancer. Exposure to ionizing radiation is linked to an increased risk of leukemia, thyroid cancer, and breast cancer.

- **EXPOSURE TO CHEMICALS AND TOXINS**

Certain chemicals and toxins, such as asbestos, benzene, and arsenic, have been linked to an increased risk of cancer. Exposure to these substances can cause DNA damage and mutations that lead to cancer.

- **AIR POLLUTION**

Exposure to outdoor air pollution has been linked to increased risk of lung cancer, bladder cancer, and other types of cancer. Indoor air pollution, including pollutants from cooking and heating fuel, has also been associated with an increased risk of cancer.

LIFESTYLE FACTORS

Lifestyle factors such as diet, exercise, and alcohol consumption can also impact cancer risk. Here are some lifestyle factors that can increase the risk of cancer:

- **POOR DIET**

A diet that is high in processed foods, red meat, and saturated fats has been linked to an increased risk of cancer. Eating a diet that is rich in fruits, vegetables, and whole grains may help reduce the risk of cancer.

- **LACK OF PHYSICAL ACTIVITY**

A sedentary lifestyle can increase the risk of many types of cancer, including breast, colon, and lung cancer. Regular physical activity has been shown to reduce the risk of cancer.

- **ALCOHOL CONSUMPTION**

Alcohol consumption has been linked to an increased risk of several types of cancer, including breast, liver, and colorectal cancer. The risk increases with the amount of alcohol consumed.

- **OBESITY**

Obesity is associated with an increased risk of several types of cancer, including breast, colon, and pancreatic cancer.

- **SMOKING**

As mentioned, smoking is a significant risk factor for cancer. Quitting smoking can reduce the risk of cancer and improve overall health.

INHERITED GENETIC MUTATIONS

Inherited genetic mutations can also increase the risk of cancer. These mutations are passed down from parent to child and can increase the likelihood of developing certain types of cancer. Here are some inherited genetic mutations that have been linked to an increased risk of cancer:

- **BRCA1 AND BRCA2 GENE MUTATIONS**

Mutations in the BRCA1 and BRCA2 genes are associated with an increased risk of breast, ovarian, and prostate cancer.

- **LYNCH SYNDROME**

Lynch Syndrome is an inherited condition that increases the risk of colorectal and other types of cancer.

- **LI-FRAUMENI SYNDROME**

Li-Fraumeni Syndrome is an inherited condition that increases the risk of several types of cancer, including breast cancer, brain tumors, and sarcomas.

- **MULTIPLE ENDOCRINE NEOPLASIA**

Multiple Endocrine Neoplasia is an inherited condition that increases the risk of several types of cancer, including thyroid, parathyroid, and adrenal gland cancer.

OTHER FACTORS

Other factors that can increase the risk of cancer include:

- **AGE**

The risk of cancer increases as a person gets older. Most cancers occur in individuals over the age of 55.

- **GENDER**

Some types of cancer are more common in men than women, such as prostate cancer. Other types of cancer, such as breast cancer, are more common in women.

- **FAMILY HISTORY**

A family history of cancer can increase the risk of developing cancer. This is because certain genetic mutations that increase the risk of cancer can be passed down from parents to children.

PART II

THE EMOTIONAL JOURNEY OF DEALING WITH CANCER

COPING WITH THE SHOCK OF CANCER DIAGNOSIS

Receiving a cancer diagnosis can be one of the most difficult and traumatic experiences of a person's life. The initial shock of the diagnosis can leave you feeling overwhelmed, scared, and confused. Coping with a cancer diagnosis is a journey that requires a combination of emotional, practical, and medical strategies. In this article, we'll explore some of the common emotions that people experience after receiving a cancer diagnosis, as well as some practical tips for coping with the shock.

First and foremost, it is important to acknowledge that a cancer diagnosis can bring up a range of emotions, from fear and anger to sadness and despair. It is completely normal to feel overwhelmed and uncertain about the future. It is important to remember that these emotions are a natural response to a difficult situation. It is important to allow yourself to feel these emotions, rather than suppressing them. Suppressing your emotions can lead to further stress and anxiety down the road. Instead, try to find healthy ways to express your emotions, such as talking to a trusted friend or family member, joining a support group, or speaking with a mental health professional.

Another important aspect of coping with a cancer diagnosis is to seek out reliable sources of information about your diagnosis and treatment options. Understanding your diagnosis and treatment options can help you feel more in control and can alleviate some of the fear and anxiety that often accompanies a cancer diagnosis. It is important to remember that not all cancers are the same, and treatment plans can vary greatly depending on the type and stage of cancer. By understanding your diagnosis, you can make informed decisions about your treatment plan and feel more empowered in the process.

Reaching out for support is another crucial aspect of coping with a cancer diagnosis. This can come in the form of family, friends, support groups, or a therapist. Talking about your diagnosis and your feelings can help you process your emotions and feel less alone. It is important to remember that seeking help is a sign of strength, not weakness. Support groups can also be a valuable resource for connecting with others who are going through a similar experience. These groups can provide a sense of community, understanding, and empathy.

Taking care of yourself is also essential during this time. Cancer treatments can take a toll on your body, both physically and emotionally. It is important to prioritize self-care activities that bring you joy and relaxation, such as reading, listening to music, or spending time in nature. Getting enough rest, eating a balanced and healthy diet, and staying physically active can also help you feel more resilient and better equipped to handle the challenges ahead.

In addition to these emotional and practical strategies, it is important to address your medical needs as well. Your medical team will play a crucial role in your cancer journey, from diagnosis to treatment and beyond. It is important to find a medical team that you trust and feel comfortable with. Ask questions and seek out second opinions if necessary. Your medical team can provide you with information about your treatment options and can help you make informed decisions about your care.

Coping with the shock of a cancer diagnosis is a journey that requires emotional, practical, and medical strategies. Remember, you are not alone in this experience and there is hope for the future. With the right mindset and support, you can face this challenge head-on, navigate the cancer journey with strength and resilience and come out stronger on the other side.

FINDING HOPE AND PURPOSE THROUGH CANCER

Cancer is a life-changing experience that can cause significant physical and emotional challenges. It is natural to feel overwhelmed and uncertain about the future when facing a cancer diagnosis. However, it is important to remember that cancer is not the end of the road. Many people who have gone through the cancer journey have found hope and purpose in their lives, even after their diagnosis. In this article, we will explore some ways to find hope and purpose through cancer.

Firstly, it is important to understand that a cancer diagnosis does not define you. It is a part of your journey, but it is not the whole story. You are still the same person you were before your diagnosis, with your own unique strengths, talents, and passions. It is important to hold on to those aspects of yourself that bring you joy and meaning, and to continue to pursue your interests and goals.

One way to find hope and purpose through cancer is to connect with others who have gone through a similar experience. Cancer support groups can be a valuable resource for connecting with others who understand what you are going through. These groups can provide a sense of community, empathy, and understanding that can help you feel less alone. You may also find inspiration and hope in hearing about the experiences and successes of others who have overcome cancer.

Another way to find hope and purpose through cancer is to focus on your personal growth and development. Cancer can be a catalyst for personal transformation, and many people have found new meaning and purpose in their lives after a cancer diagnosis. This may involve exploring new interests, developing new skills, or pursuing new career opportunities. By focusing on personal growth and development, you can find new ways to contribute to the world and make a positive impact on others.

In addition to personal growth, finding meaning through service can also be a powerful way to cope with cancer. This may involve volunteering at a cancer center or hospital, participating in cancer fundraising events, or advocating for cancer research and treatment. By giving back to others, you can find a sense of purpose and fulfillment, and can make a meaningful difference in the lives of others.

Finally, finding hope and purpose through cancer may also involve spiritual or religious practices. Many people find comfort and strength in their faith during difficult times, and cancer can be an opportunity to deepen your spiritual connection and explore new ways of understanding the world. This may involve exploring new religious or spiritual practices, connecting with a spiritual community, or finding comfort and inspiration in prayer or meditation.

Fnding hope and purpose through cancer is possible, even in the face of a challenging diagnosis. By focusing on personal growth, connecting with others, giving back through service, and exploring spiritual practices, you can find new ways to thrive and make a positive impact on the world. Remember that cancer is just one part of your journey, and that you are still the same unique and valuable person you were before your diagnosis. By embracing your strengths, passions, and interests, you can find new ways to bring hope and purpose to your life and to others.

SEEKING MEDICAL TREATMENT AND SUPPORT

Seeking medical treatment and support is essential when facing a cancer diagnosis. The earlier the cancer is detected and treated, the better the chances of survival and recovery. In this article, we will explore the importance of seeking medical treatment and support, and some tips for finding the right healthcare team.

The first step in seeking medical treatment and support is to find a healthcare team that you trust and feel comfortable with. This may involve consulting with your primary care physician or getting referrals from friends, family members, or cancer support groups. When looking for a healthcare team, it is important to consider factors such as experience, expertise, and communication skills. You should feel confident that your healthcare team has the knowledge and skills necessary to provide you with the best possible care, and that they are able to communicate effectively with you and your loved ones.

Once you have found a healthcare team, it is important to work with them to develop a treatment plan that is tailored to your specific needs and preferences. This may involve undergoing diagnostic tests such as imaging scans, biopsies, or blood tests to determine the type and stage of your cancer. Based on these results, your healthcare team will develop a treatment plan that may involve surgery, chemotherapy, radiation therapy, or a combination of these treatments. It is important to ask questions and express your concerns or preferences throughout this process, and to work closely with your healthcare team to make informed decisions about your treatment options.

In addition to medical treatment, it is important to seek emotional support to help you cope with the challenges of cancer. Many cancer centers offer support groups, counseling services, and other resources to help patients and their families manage the emotional impact of cancer. You may also find support from friends and family members or through online communities and forums.

It is also very important to take care of your physical health during cancer treatment as well. This may involve making changes to your diet and exercise routine, getting enough rest, and managing any side effects of treatment. Your healthcare team can provide guidance on how to manage side effects such as nausea, fatigue, and pain.

Managing the financial aspects of cancer treatment can also be a challenge. It is important to understand your insurance coverage and to talk to your healthcare team about any financial concerns you may have. Many cancer centers offer financial assistance programs and can help you navigate the insurance and billing process.

Finally, it is important to take an active role in your cancer treatment and to advocate for yourself. This may involve asking questions, seeking second opinions, and communicating your needs and concerns to your healthcare team. By being an active participant in your treatment, you can feel more empowered and in control of your cancer diagnosis.

In conclusion, seeking medical treatment and support is an important part of coping with a cancer diagnosis. By finding a healthcare team that you trust, being informed about your treatment options, seeking emotional support, taking care of your physical health, managing the financial aspects of treatment, and advocating for yourself, you can feel more in control of your cancer diagnosis and can improve your overall quality of life. Remember that you are not alone in this journey and that there are resources available to help you every step of the way.

PART III

THE PHYSICAL JOURNEY OF DEALING WITH CANCER

CANCER TREATMENT OPTIONS

When someone receives a cancer diagnosis, one of the first questions that comes to mind is usually, "What are my treatment options?" The answer depends on several factors, including the type and stage of cancer, as well as the patient's overall health and medical history.

There are several types of cancer treatment, including surgery, chemotherapy, radiation therapy, immunotherapy, targeted therapy, and hormone therapy. Your healthcare team will work with you to develop a treatment plan that is tailored to your specific needs and goals.

SURGERY

Surgery is often the first line of treatment for many types of cancer. The goal of surgery is to remove the cancerous tumor from the body. There are several types of surgery used to treat cancer, including:

Curative Surgery: This is used to remove the entire tumor or cancerous tissue from the body, and it is often used when cancer is detected at an early stage.

Preventive Surgery: This is used to remove tissue that is not cancerous but has a high risk of becoming cancerous in the future, such as a benign tumor.

Palliative Surgery: This is used to reduce pain and other symptoms associated with cancer, but it is not intended to cure the disease.

The benefits of surgery include:

- **Can be efficiently curative:** Surgery can often remove the cancerous tissue completely and cure the patient of cancer.
- **Aids in determining the extent of the cancer:** Surgery can also be used to biopsy the cancerous tissue to help determine the extent of the cancer and whether further treatment is necessary.
- **Relieves symptoms:** Surgery can be used to relieve pain and other symptoms associated with the cancer.

Potential side effects of surgery include:

- **Pain and discomfort:** Patients may experience pain and discomfort after surgery, which can be managed with pain medication.
- **Infection:** Surgery can increase the risk of infection, which can be prevented with antibiotics.
- **Scarring:** Surgery can leave a visible scar, although plastic surgery techniques can often minimize scarring.

CHEMOTHERAPY

Chemotherapy uses drugs to kill cancer cells. The drugs can be given orally or through injection, and they travel throughout the body to reach cancer cells. Chemotherapy can be used alone or in combination with other treatments, such as surgery or radiation therapy.

The benefits of chemotherapy include:

- **Can be used in combination with other treatments:** Chemotherapy can be used in combination with surgery or radiation therapy to increase effectiveness.
- **Helps prevent recurrence:** Chemotherapy can be used to prevent cancer from coming back.

Potential side effects:

- **Nausea and vomiting:** Chemotherapy can cause nausea and vomiting, which can be managed with medication.
- **Hair loss:** Chemotherapy can cause hair loss, although it often grows back after treatment.
- **Weakened immune system:** Chemotherapy can weaken the immune system, making patients more susceptible to infection.

RADIATION THERAPY

Radiation therapy uses high-energy radiation to kill cancer cells. It can be used alone or in combination with other cancer treatments, such as surgery or chemotherapy. There are two types of radiation therapy:

External Beam Radiation Therapy: This type of radiation is delivered from a machine outside the body.

Internal Radiation Therapy (Brachytherapy): This type of radiation is delivered directly to the tumor through a catheter or implant.

The benefits of radiation therapy include:

- **Effectively curative:** Radiation therapy can often be used as a primary treatment to cure cancer.
- **Can be used in combination with other** treatments: Radiation therapy can be used in combination with surgery or chemotherapy to increase effectiveness.

Potential side effects of radiation therapy:

- **Fatigue:** Patients may experience fatigue during and after radiation therapy, which can be managed with rest.

- **Skin changes:** Radiation therapy can cause skin changes such as redness, dryness, and peeling.
- **Radiation sickness:** Patients may experience nausea, vomiting, and diarrhea during and after radiation therapy.

IMMUNOTHERAPY

Immunotherapy is a type of cancer treatment that works by stimulating the immune system to attack cancer cells. This type of treatment is often used to treat melanoma, lung cancer, and bladder cancer.

The benefits of immunotherapy include:

- **Long-lasting response:** Immunotherapy can provide a long-lasting response, with some patients experiencing remission for several years.
- **Effective in some cases:** Immunotherapy can be effective in some cases where other treatments have failed.

Potential side effects of immunotherapy include:

- **Fatigue:** This is the most common side effect of immunotherapy and can be managed with rest and lifestyle changes.
- **Skin problems:** Immunotherapy can cause skin problems, such as rash and itching.

- **Gastrointestinal problems:** Immunotherapy can cause gastrointestinal problems, such as diarrhea and nausea.

TARGETED THERAPY

Targeted therapy is a type of cancer treatment that uses drugs to target specific molecules involved in cancer cell growth and survival. This type of treatment is often used to treat lung cancer, breast cancer, and colorectal cancer.

The benefits of targeted therapy include:

- **More effective in some cases:** Targeted therapy can be more effective than chemotherapy in some cases, especially in cancers that have specific genetic mutations.
- **More personalized treatment:** Targeted therapy can be tailored to the specific molecular characteristics of a patient's cancer.

Potential side effects of targeted therapy include:

- **Skin problems:** Targeted therapy can cause skin problems, such as rash and dry skin.
- **Gastrointestinal problems:** Targeted therapy can cause gastrointestinal problems, such as diarrhea and nausea.

- **Cardiovascular problems:** Targeted therapy can cause cardiovascular problems, such as high blood pressure and heart failure.

HORMONE THERAPY

Hormone therapy is a type of cancer treatment that works by either blocking the production of certain hormones or preventing them from acting on cancer cells. This type of treatment is often used to treat breast cancer, prostate cancer, and ovarian cancer.

The benefits of hormone therapy include:

- **Reduced risk of cancer recurrence:** Hormone therapy can reduce the risk of cancer recurrence by up to 50% in patients with hormone-sensitive cancers.
- **Effective in combination with other treatments:** Hormone therapy can be used in combination with other treatments, such as radiation therapy, to increase effectiveness.

Potential side effects of hormone therapy include:

- **Hot flashes:** This is the most common side effect of hormone therapy and can be managed with medication or lifestyle changes.

- **Mood changes:** Hormone therapy can cause mood changes, such as depression and anxiety.
- **Bone loss:** Hormone therapy can lead to bone loss, increasing the risk of osteoporosis.

It's important to remember that every cancer diagnosis is unique and that there is no one-size-fits-all approach to treatment. Your healthcare team will work with you to develop a treatment plan that is tailored to your specific needs and goals. It's important to ask questions, seek second opinions, and be an active participant in your treatment. By working closely with your healthcare team, you can feel more in control of your cancer diagnosis and improve your overall quality of life.

COPING WITH THE SIDE EFFECTS OF CANCER TREATMENT

Coping with the side effects of cancer treatment can be challenging, but it is an essential part of the journey towards recovery. The side effects of treatment can vary depending on the type of cancer, the stage of the disease, and the treatment method used. It's important to understand that not everyone experiences the same side effects, and the severity of the side effects can also vary. Coping with these side effects requires a multifaceted approach that involves both medical and non-medical interventions. Here are some tips to help you cope with the most common side effects of cancer treatment.

COPING WITH FATIGUE

Fatigue is one of the most common side effects of cancer treatment, and it can be one of the most challenging to manage. Coping with fatigue requires a multi-pronged approach that involves both rest and activity. It's essential to listen to your body and take rest breaks when needed. However, it's also essential to stay active and engage in light exercise, such as walking, yoga, or swimming. Exercise can help boost energy levels and reduce fatigue. Other strategies that can help manage fatigue include getting adequate sleep, eating a healthy diet, and reducing stress through relaxation techniques such as meditation or deep breathing.

COPING WITH NAUSEA AND VOMITING

Nausea and vomiting are common side effects of chemotherapy and radiation therapy. Coping with these side effects requires a combination of medication and lifestyle changes. Anti-nausea medications prescribed by your doctor can help reduce the severity of these side effects. Eating small, frequent meals and avoiding foods that trigger nausea, such as spicy or greasy foods, can also be helpful. Drinking plenty of fluids, such as water, herbal tea, or clear broths, can also help prevent dehydration.

COPING WITH HAIR LOSS

Hair loss is a common side effect of chemotherapy, and it can be emotionally distressing for many people. Coping with hair loss requires a combination of practical and emotional strategies. Wearing a wig or a scarf can help cover hair loss and boost confidence. Some people choose to shave their heads to take control of the hair loss process. Others may find solace in support groups or counseling to help manage the emotional impact of hair loss.

COPING WITH SKIN CHANGES

Skin changes, such as dryness, itching, and rashes, are common side effects of cancer treatment. Coping with these side effects requires a combination of medical and non-medical interventions. Moisturizing your skin regularly with fragrance-free lotions or creams can help prevent dryness and itching. Wearing loose-fitting clothing made of breathable fabrics, such as cotton or linen, can also help reduce irritation. Some people may require prescription creams or ointments to manage more severe skin changes.

COPING WITH PAIN

Pain is a common side effect of cancer treatment, and it can be both physical and emotional. Coping with pain requires a combination of medication and non-medication interventions. Pain medications prescribed by your doctor can help manage physical pain. However, non-medication interventions such as relaxation techniques, massage, or acupuncture can also be helpful in reducing pain. Counseling or therapy can also help manage emotional pain and provide coping strategies to deal with chronic pain.

COPING WITH NEUROPATHY

Neuropathy is a side effect of chemotherapy that can cause numbness, tingling, or weakness in the hands and feet. Coping with neuropathy requires a combination of medication and lifestyle changes. Medications such as gabapentin or pregabalin can help manage the symptoms of neuropathy. Engaging in light exercise, such as walking or swimming, can also help reduce neuropathy symptoms. Wearing supportive shoes and avoiding tight socks or stockings can also help reduce the severity of neuropathy.

COPING WITH EMOTIONAL AND MENTAL HEALTH CHANGES

Cancer can be a devastating diagnosis that can affect not only physical health but also emotional and mental well-being. The emotional and mental impact of cancer can be just as significant as the physical effects, and it's important to prioritize your mental health and emotional well-being throughout your cancer journey. Coping with emotional and mental health changes is an important part of cancer treatment, and there are many strategies and resources available to help you navigate this aspect of your cancer journey.

The emotional and mental health challenges that come with a cancer diagnosis can vary from person to person and may include anxiety, depression, stress, fear, and uncertainty. Coping with these challenges can be difficult, but it's important to remember that you are not alone. Many cancer patients and survivors have experienced these same emotions and have found ways to cope and move forward.

One strategy for coping with emotional and mental health changes is to seek support. This can come in many forms, including talking to loved ones, joining a support group, or working with a therapist. Support can be a valuable resource for coping with the emotional and mental challenges of cancer, providing a safe space to share your feelings and experiences and helping you to feel less alone.

Another strategy for coping with emotional and mental health changes is to take care of yourself physically. Eating a healthy diet, getting enough sleep, and engaging in regular physical activity can all help to improve your mental well-being. Additionally, participating in relaxation techniques such as meditation, yoga, or tai chi can be helpful in reducing stress and anxiety.

It's also important to practice Self-compassion during your cancer journey. Cancer treatment can be difficult and overwhelming, and it's important to remember that you are doing the best you can. Don't be too hard on yourself and take time to acknowledge the progress you are making, no matter how small.

Cancer can also have a significant impact on relationships with family and friends, and it's important to communicate with your loved ones about your emotional and mental health. Let them know how you are feeling and what they can do to support you. Additionally, it's important to set boundaries and prioritize your own needs, even if that means saying no to certain requests or invitations.

Finally, it's important to stay engaged in activities that bring you joy and purpose. This may include hobbies, volunteering, or spending time with loved ones. These activities can provide a sense of meaning and purpose during a difficult time and can help to improve your emotional and mental well-being.

In addition to these strategies, there are also many resources available to help cancer patients and survivors cope with emotional and mental health changes. Cancer support organizations, offer a variety of resources, including support groups, counseling, and educational materials. Additionally, many hospitals and cancer treatment centers offer counseling services or referrals to mental health professionals.

Coping with emotional and mental health changes is an important aspect of cancer treatment. By seeking support, taking care of yourself physically, communicating with loved ones, staying engaged in activities that bring you joy and purpose, and utilizing available resources, you can navigate the emotional and mental challenges of cancer and move forward with hope and resilience.

PART IV

LIFESTYLE CHANGES

A HOLISTIC APPROACH TO RECOVERY

A cancer diagnosis is an event that can have a significant impact on a person's physical, emotional, and spiritual well-being. While medical treatments such as chemotherapy, radiation, and surgery are often necessary to fight cancer, they can also take a toll on the body and mind. That's why many cancer survivors and healthcare professionals advocate for a holistic approach to recovery that addresses the whole person, not just their cancer.

A holistic approach to cancer recovery recognizes that the body, mind, and spirit are interconnected and that treating the whole person is essential to achieving optimal health and well-being. This approach takes into account a person's physical, emotional, and spiritual needs and seeks to support and enhance their overall health and resilience. Here are some of the key components of a holistic approach to recovery for cancer survivors:

NUTRITION AND EXERCISE

Good nutrition and regular exercise are essential for maintaining a healthy body and mind, especially during and after cancer treatment. A balanced diet that includes plenty of fruits, vegetables, whole grains, and lean protein can help boost the immune system and improve energy levels. Exercise can help reduce fatigue, improve mood, and increase physical strength and endurance. Many cancer survivors find that activities such as yoga, tai chi, or walking in nature can be particularly beneficial for their overall well-being.

MIND-BODY PRACTICES

Mind-body practices such as meditation, deep breathing, and visualization can help reduce stress and anxiety, improve sleep, and promote relaxation. These practices can also help cancer survivors cope with the emotional and psychological challenges of cancer treatment and recovery. Some cancer survivors may also benefit from therapies such as acupuncture, massage, or chiropractic care to help alleviate pain and promote relaxation.

SUPPORTIVE RELATIONSHIPS

Having a strong support network of family, friends, and healthcare professionals can be crucial for cancer survivors. Supportive relationships can provide emotional and practical support, reduce stress and anxiety, and improve overall well-being. Joining a cancer support group or connecting with other survivors can also help reduce feelings of isolation and provide a sense of community.

SPIRITUAL AND EMOTIONAL WELLNESS

Cancer can be a deeply spiritual and emotional experience for many people. Exploring one's spirituality or engaging in activities that promote emotional well-being, such as journaling or creative expression, can be helpful for some cancer survivors. Others may find solace in religious or spiritual practices, such as prayer or attending church. Seeking professional counseling or therapy can also be beneficial for those struggling with the emotional challenges of cancer.

SELF-CARE

Self-care is an essential component of a holistic approach to cancer recovery. Taking time to rest, engage in enjoyable activities, and prioritize one's own needs can help reduce stress and promote overall well-being. Practicing self-compassion and self-acceptance can also help cancer survivors cope with the physical and emotional changes that may accompany cancer treatment.

Incorporating these five components into a cancer survivor's recovery plan can help promote overall health and well-being. However, it's important to remember that everyone's journey is unique, and what works for one person may not work for another. It's essential to work with healthcare professionals and trusted support networks to develop an individualized approach to recovery that meets a person's specific needs and goals.

A holistic approach to cancer recovery recognizes the interconnectedness of the body, mind, and spirit and seeks to support and enhance a person's overall well-being.

NUTRITION AND CANCER: EATING FOR HEALTH

Nutrition plays a vital role in cancer prevention and treatment. Eating a well-balanced diet can help cancer patients to feel better, manage symptoms, and tolerate cancer treatments. This article will discuss the importance of nutrition in cancer care and recommend various healthy foods to eat during and after cancer treatment.

Poor nutrition is a common problem among cancer patients. Many cancer treatments can cause unpleasant side effects, such as nausea, vomiting, and diarrhea. These side effects can lead to loss of appetite, decreased food intake, and malnutrition. Cancer patients who are malnourished are more likely to experience complications, such as infections, slower healing, and reduced quality of life.

One of the most important things for cancer patients to remember is to consume enough calories and protein to maintain their weight, muscle mass, and strength. A high protein diet that includes plenty of lean meats, fish, poultry, beans, and nuts can help with muscle recovery after cancer treatment.

Eating a variety of fruits and vegetables is also crucial for cancer patients. Fruits and vegetables are packed with vitamins, minerals, and antioxidants that help fight cancer cells and reduce inflammation. Leafy greens, such as spinach, kale, and collard greens, are particularly nutrient-dense and should be consumed regularly.

Cancer patients should also avoid or limit their intake of foods that may increase their risk of cancer or worsen their condition. These foods include processed meats, sugar-sweetened beverages, trans fats, and high-fat foods, such as fried foods, baked goods, and fatty meats.

The following are some recommendations for healthy foods to eat during and after cancer treatment:

- **WHOLE GRAINS**

Whole grains are a good source of fiber, which can help regulate digestion and prevent constipation, a common side effect of cancer treatment. Whole grains also contain many nutrients, such as B vitamins, iron, and magnesium, that can help cancer patients stay healthy.

Examples of whole grains include quinoa, brown rice, whole-grain bread, and oatmeal.

- **LEAN PROTEIN**

Protein is necessary for muscle recovery and can help cancer patients regain their strength after treatment. Lean protein sources, such as chicken, fish, turkey, and plant-based proteins like beans or tofu are great sources of protein.

- **FRUITS AND VEGETABLES**

Fruits and vegetables are packed with vitamins, minerals, and antioxidants that help fight cancer cells and reduce inflammation. Dark, leafy greens, such as spinach, kale, and collard greens are particularly nutrient-dense and should be consumed regularly.

- **HEALTHY FATS**

Healthy fats, including omega-3 fatty acids and monounsaturated fats, can help reduce inflammation and promote heart health. Examples of healthy fats include fatty fish like salmon, nuts, seeds, and oils like olive oil.

- **FERMENTED FOODS**

Fermented foods contain probiotics, which can promote gut health and boost the immune system.

Examples of fermented foods include kefir, yogurt, kimchi, and sauerkraut.

In addition to eating a healthy diet, cancer patients should also stay hydrated by drinking plenty of water, avoiding sugary drinks and alcohol, and getting enough rest and exercise.

While a healthy diet can help prevent and manage cancer, it's important to remember that no single food or nutrient can cure cancer on its own. Cancer treatment may require a specialized diet, and it's important to talk to a doctor or dietitian before making any significant changes to your diet.

However, by making healthy food choices, cancer patients can improve their overall health and quality of life, which can help them more effectively manage their cancer diagnosis and treatment.

In summary, nutrition is a vital component of cancer treatment and prevention. A healthy diet can help cancer patients manage side effects, fight cancer cells, and maintain their overall health and well-being. It's important for cancer patients to work with their healthcare team to develop a personalized nutrition plan that meets their specific needs and goals.

EXERCISE AND CANCER: MOVING TOWARD WELLNESS

Exercise is an essential component of a healthy lifestyle, and it's especially important for people who are living with cancer. Engaging in regular physical activity can help cancer survivors manage the physical and emotional side effects of treatment, improve their overall health and well-being, and reduce the risk of cancer recurrence. In this chapter, we'll explore the benefits of exercise for cancer survivors and provide practical tips for incorporating physical activity into your daily routine.

THE BENEFITS OF EXERCISE FOR CANCER PATIENTS AND SURVIVORS

Cancer treatment can take a toll on the body, causing fatigue, muscle weakness, and other physical symptoms. However, research has shown that exercise can help reduce these symptoms, improve physical function, and enhance quality of life for people with cancer. Here are some of the benefits of exercise for cancer survivors:

- **Reducing fatigue:** Exercise can help combat cancer-related fatigue, which is one of the most common and distressing side effects of cancer treatment. Regular physical activity has been shown to improve energy levels and reduce feelings of tiredness.

- **Improving strength and mobility:** Cancer treatment can cause muscle weakness and loss of flexibility, which can make it difficult to perform everyday activities. Exercise can help improve strength, flexibility, and mobility, making it easier to perform daily tasks and enjoy leisure activities.

- **Enhancing mental health:** Cancer can take a toll on a person's emotional well-being, leading to feelings of anxiety, depression, and stress. Exercise has been shown to have a positive impact on mental health, reducing symptoms of anxiety and depression and improving overall mood.

- **Reducing the risk of recurrence:** Exercise has been shown to reduce the risk of cancer recurrence in people with breast, colon, and other types of cancer. Regular physical activity can help improve immune function and reduce inflammation, which are factors that can contribute to cancer growth and recurrence.

TIPS FOR INCORPORATING EXERCISE INTO YOUR ROUTINE

If you're a cancer survivor, it's important to talk to your healthcare team before starting an exercise program. They can help you determine what types of exercise are safe and appropriate for your individual needs and abilities. Here are some tips for incorporating exercise into your routine:

- **Start Slowly:** If you're not used to regular physical activity, start with low-intensity exercises such as walking, gentle yoga or stretching. Gradually increase the intensity and duration of your workouts as you build strength and stamina.

- **Find an exercise buddy:** Exercising with a friend or family member can make it more enjoyable and help keep you motivated. Consider joining a cancer support group or exercise class designed specifically for cancer survivors.

- **Mix it up:** Variety is key to staying motivated and avoiding boredom. Try different types of exercise, such as swimming, cycling, or strength training, to keep your workouts interesting.

- **Set realistic goals:** Setting achievable goals can help you stay motivated and track your progress. Start with small, achievable goals and gradually increase the challenge as you build strength and stamina.

- **Listen to your body:** Pay attention to how your body feels during and after exercise. If you experience pain, dizziness, or other symptoms, slow down or stop exercising and talk to your healthcare team.

- **Make it a habit:** Consistency is key to reaping the benefits of exercise. Aim for at least 150 minutes of moderate-intensity exercise per week or 75 minutes of vigorous-intensity exercise per week.

SLEEP, STRESS, AND OTHER LIFESTYLE FACTORS

When it comes to cancer treatment and survival, there are many factors that can impact the outcome. While medical treatment is essential, there are also lifestyle factors that can play a significant role in supporting the body's ability to heal and recover. Some of the most important lifestyle factors to consider are sleep, stress, and other lifestyle habits.

SLEEP

Getting enough sleep is essential for overall health, but it is especially important for cancer survivors. Sleep helps the body repair and regenerate tissues, and it plays a crucial role in immune function. Lack of sleep can lead to fatigue, which is a common side effect of cancer treatment, and can make it more difficult for the body to fight off infections.

It is recommended that adults get between 7-9 hours of sleep per night. However, cancer survivors may need even more sleep to support their recovery. If you are experiencing fatigue or difficulty sleeping, talk to your healthcare provider. They may be able to suggest strategies for improving your sleep, such as establishing a regular sleep schedule, avoiding caffeine and alcohol before bedtime, and creating a relaxing bedtime routine.

STRESS

Stress is a normal part of life, but too much stress can have negative effects on the body. Chronic stress can lead to inflammation and weaken the immune system, which can make it more difficult for the body to fight off cancer and other illnesses.

Cancer diagnosis and treatment can be incredibly stressful, but there are ways to manage stress and reduce its impact on the body. Some strategies that may be helpful include:

- Mind-body practices such as meditation, yoga, and tai chi.
- Exercise, which can help reduce stress and improve overall health.
- Talking to a therapist or counselor, who can provide support and strategies for coping with stress.
- Connecting with friends and family, which can provide emotional support and a sense of community

OTHER LIFESTYLE FACTORS

In addition to sleep and stress, there are other lifestyle factors that can impact cancer survival. Some of these include:

DIET

Eating a healthy diet that is rich in fruits, vegetables, whole grains, and lean protein can help support the body's ability to heal and recover. It is also important to stay hydrated by drinking plenty of water and other fluids.

SMOKING AND ALCOHOL USE

Smoking and excessive alcohol use can increase the risk of cancer recurrence and other health problems. If you smoke or drink alcohol, talk to your healthcare provider about strategies for quitting or reducing your use.

SUN EXPOSURE

Exposure to the sun's harmful UV rays can increase the risk of skin cancer. It is important to protect your skin by wearing sunscreen, protective clothing, and seeking shade when possible.

It is important to remember that making lifestyle changes can be challenging, especially during cancer treatment and recovery. It is okay to start small and make gradual changes over time. It can also be helpful to enlist the support of friends, family, and healthcare providers to help you stay on track and make positive changes.

Sleep, stress, and other lifestyle factors can play a significant role in cancer survival. By prioritizing healthy habits and making positive lifestyle changes, cancer survivors can support their body's ability to heal and recover. It is important to work with healthcare providers to develop a comprehensive plan for overall health and well-being, including medical treatment, lifestyle changes, and other support resources.

PROVIDING SELF-CARE DURING RECOVERY

One of the most crucial aspects of cancer recovery is self-care. Cancer treatment takes a toll on the body, and the recovery process can be exhausting, both physically and emotionally. However, taking steps to care for oneself can greatly improve the recovery process and lead to a better quality of life.

The first step in self-care during recovery is to ensure that one is getting enough rest. Rest is essential, and the body will need more than usual during the recovery process. It is important to remember that rest does not just mean sleep – incorporating relaxation and meditation techniques can also be beneficial. Taking breaks throughout the day to relax, breathe deeply, or meditate can help to reduce stress levels, which can in turn improve sleep quality and promote overall well-being.

Another critical form of self-care during recovery is diet and nutrition as already mentioned. It is crucial to maintain a healthy diet, which should be high in protein, fruits, and vegetables. A healthy diet can help to provide the body with the nutrients it needs to heal and fight off any infections. It is also essential to stay hydrated by drinking plenty of Water, particularly after chemotherapy or radiation treatments, which can cause dehydration.

In addition to diet and rest, maintaining an active lifestyle can help to improve overall well-being during the recovery process. Exercise has been shown to lower stress levels, increase energy levels, and promote better sleep quality. It is important to note that exercise should be moderate and tailored to the individual's needs and abilities, particularly during the recovery process.

Aside from physical self-care, it is also important to address mental and emotional self-care during recovery. Cancer treatment can take a toll on one's mental health, leading to depression, anxiety, and other psychological challenges. It can be helpful to seek out support groups and counseling to help cope with the emotional challenges that come with cancer treatment. Additionally, incorporating activities such as journaling, meditation, or other mindfulness practices can help to reduce stress and improve overall mental health.

Another essential aspect of self-care during recovery is attending regular medical appointments and following medication schedules. It is important to work closely with one's healthcare team to ensure that treatments are effective and side effects are managed properly. Following medication schedules and attending regular appointments can help to prevent any complications and ensure a successful recovery.

Finally, it is important to remember that self-care is not a one-size-fits-all approach. What works for one person may not work for another, and it is important to listen to one's body and needs. It is essential to find a self-care routine that works for you and incorporates activities that you enjoy and find beneficial.

SUPPORT SYSTEMS

No one should ever have to go through cancer alone. This is where support systems come in. Support systems are essential for cancer survivors to help them navigate the challenges of diagnosis, treatment, and recovery.

A support system can consist of family, friends, healthcare providers, support groups, and other resources. These individuals and groups can provide emotional support, practical assistance, and valuable information to help cancer survivors and their families cope with the physical, emotional, and practical challenges of cancer.

EMOTIONAL SUPPORT

Emotional support is one of the most important aspects of a support system. Cancer can take a toll on a person's mental health and emotional well-being, and having a network of people to lean on can make all the difference. A supportive friend or family member can provide a listening ear, words of encouragement, and a sense of normalcy during a difficult time. Support groups can also be a valuable resource for emotional support, as they provide a safe space for individuals to share their experiences and connect with others who understand what they are going through.

PRACTICAL ASSISTANCE

Practical assistance can also be an essential part of a support system. During cancer treatment, individuals may experience physical limitations or side effects that make it difficult to perform daily tasks. Friends and family members can provide practical assistance such as cooking meals, running errands, and helping with household chores. Healthcare providers can also offer practical assistance by connecting patients with resources such as transportation to appointments, financial assistance programs, and home healthcare services.

INFORMATION AND RESOURCES

Information and resources are another important aspect of a support system. Cancer treatment can be complex, and having access to accurate information and helpful resources can help individuals make informed decisions about their care. Healthcare providers can provide information about treatment options, side effects, and managing symptoms. Support groups and online forums can also be a valuable resource for information and advice from others who have gone through similar experiences.

Support systems are essential for cancer survivors and their families. Emotional support, practical assistance, and information and resources can help individuals navigate the challenges of cancer treatment and recovery. It is important for cancer survivors to reach out to loved ones, healthcare providers, and support groups to build a strong support system that will help them through their cancer journey. No one should ever have to go through cancer alone, and with a strong support system in place, cancer survivors can take on the challenges of their journey with hope and strength.

BUILDING YOUR HEALTHCARE TEAM

Building your healthcare team, which includes medical professionals, family, and friends, can help you manage the physical, emotional, and mental impacts of cancer treatment. These support systems can provide different types of support that can help you through difficult times and keep you on track with your cancer treatment.

When building your healthcare team, start with your medical professionals. This includes your oncologist, surgeon, primary care physician, and other healthcare providers who are involved in your treatment plan. These individuals are your primary source of information about your diagnosis, treatment options, and potential side effects. You should feel comfortable asking questions and discussing your concerns with them. They should also be able to provide you with resources to help you manage side effects and help you make decisions about your treatment options.

It is also essential to take care of your emotional and mental wellbeing during your treatment journey. Consider seeking the help of a mental health professional, such as a therapist or counselor, who can offer support with any anxiety, depression, or other emotional concerns. They can also help you manage stress and cope with the changes in your life.

Finally, it is important to take care of your physical health during treatment. Consider building a team of healthcare providers that emphasize your overall wellbeing, such as a nutritionist, physical therapist or fitness coach. These professionals can help you develop an exercise routine and provide guidance on how to make dietary changes to help manage cancer-related symptoms.

In summary, building your healthcare team is essential when it comes to cancer treatment and recovery.

These support systems can provide different types of support that can help you manage the physical, emotional, and mental impacts of cancer treatment. Remember to communicate openly with your team and advocate for yourself to ensure that you have the best possible support throughout your cancer journey.

NAVIGATING RELATIONSHIPS WITH FAMILY AND FRIENDS

Getting support from your family and friends is an essential aspect of the cancer journey. Cancer can be a life-altering experience, both physically and emotionally, and having a support system of family and friends can make all the difference in coping with the challenges that arise.

First and foremost, it is important to communicate your needs and feelings with your loved ones. Open and honest communication is key to maintaining healthy relationships during this difficult time. It is important to remember that your loved ones may be experiencing their own emotions and reactions to your diagnosis, so it is crucial to create a space where everyone can share their thoughts and feelings without judgment.

It is also important to set boundaries and ask for help when needed. Cancer treatment can be physically and emotionally exhausting, and it is okay to ask for assistance with daily tasks or emotional support. This may include help with household chores, transportation to appointments, or simply someone to listen and provide comfort.

Maintaining social connections can also be beneficial for mental and emotional well-being. While cancer treatment may require some changes to your social life, it is important to stay connected with friends and family. This can include scheduling social outings or activities that are manageable within your treatment plan, or connecting with others who have experienced cancer through support groups or online communities.

It is also important to address any conflicts or issues that may arise within relationships. Cancer can bring up a range of emotions, including fear, anger, and frustration, and it is important to address any conflicts in a constructive and respectful manner. This may involve seeking the help of a therapist or counselor to mediate discussions and provide support.

Finally, it is important to prioritize self-care and maintain a sense of normalcy as much as possible. This may involve engaging in activities that bring joy and relaxation, such as yoga, meditation, or creative hobbies. It may also involve setting boundaries around work or other obligations to prioritize rest and recovery.

By prioritizing communication, setting boundaries, maintaining social connections, addressing conflicts, and prioritizing self-care, you can build a strong support system that will help you through this difficult time.

JOINING A SUPPORT GROUP

For cancer survivors, joining a support group can be an important step in creating a strong support system. A support group can provide emotional support, information, and resources to help those who have gone through cancer feel less alone and more empowered. In this chapter, we will explore the benefits of joining a support group, as well as some tips for finding the right group for you.

BENEFITS OF JOINING A SUPPORT GROUP

One of the primary benefits of joining a support group for cancer survivors is the emotional support that it provides. Cancer can be a lonely and isolating experience, especially when friends and family members can't fully understand what you're going through. A support group offers a safe space to share your thoughts and feelings with others who have gone through similar experiences.

Another benefit of joining a support group is access to information and resources. Cancer can be overwhelming, and it can be difficult to navigate the healthcare system and find the support that you need. A support group can provide information about treatment options, clinical trials, and other resources that may be helpful.

TIPS FOR FINDING THE RIGHT SUPPORT GROUP

When looking for a support group, it's important to find one that meets your needs. Here are some tips for finding the right group:

- Ask your healthcare team for recommendations. They may be able to recommend a support group that is specifically for cancer survivors.

- Look for groups that focus on your particular type of cancer. Different types of cancer may require different treatment and support, so finding a group that is specific to your type of cancer can be helpful.

- Attend a few meetings before deciding if a group is right for you. It's important to find a group where you feel comfortable and supported.

- Consider joining an online support group. Online groups can be a great option for those who may not have access to local groups or prefer to connect with others from the comfort of their own home.

Joining a support group can be a valuable source of emotional support, information, and resources for cancer survivors. By finding the right group and connecting with others who have gone through similar experiences, survivors can feel less alone and more empowered as they navigate the challenges of cancer.

PART V

MOVING FORWARD

FINDING MEANING AND PURPOSE

For anyone who has experienced the devastating diagnosis of cancer, it can be easy to feel lost and adrift in a sea of uncertainty. Suddenly, life as you knew it is turned upside-down, and the future becomes uncertain. In the midst of this turmoil, finding meaning and purpose can seem like an impossible task. But it is precisely during these challenging times that we most need to discover our sense of purpose, to rediscover what gives our lives meaning and fulfillment.

The journey of healing and recovery from cancer is a transformative one, and the experience can leave survivors with newfound purpose and drive. It's crucial to focus on the positive aspects of this life-altering experience to find meaning and purpose in the aftermath.

One way to start this process is by examining your priorities and values. Reflecting on what is truly important to you can help guide you towards finding meaning and purpose. For instance, if family is important to you, you may choose to spend more time with loved ones and make the most of meaningful connections.

Survivors can also develop a sense of purpose through community involvement, which can also provide a sense of fulfillment. Volunteering with cancer organizations or participating in charity events can be a great way to give back and make a change in the lives of other survivors.

Another way to find meaning and purpose is to explore new hobbies or interests. Engaging in activities that bring you joy can help you rediscover your passions and create a renewed sense of purpose. Also, sharing your story can help others and give you a sense of purpose while spreading awareness about the realities of cancer.

Finding meaning and purpose after surviving cancer is a unique and individual journey. Whether it's through reflecting on values, community involvement, pursuing new hobbies and interests, or sharing your story, it's important to focus on the positive aspects of the experience to create a sense of purpose and fulfillment. Through this process, survivors can learn to appreciate their newfound perspective and find joy and purpose in life after cancer.

FINDING HOPE AND INSPIRATION IN YOUR JOURNEY

Cancer patients can experience a range of emotions such as anxiety, fear, grief, and even depression, which can be detrimental to their health. Therefore, seeking hope and inspiration can help patients stay positive and improve their quality of life.

There are several ways cancer patients can find hope and inspiration in their journey. Firstly, joining a support group can be beneficial. Sharing experiences with others who have gone through similar situations can provide comfort and reassurance. Support groups can help patients feel less isolated and more supported, which can help them find the strength to persevere through tough times.

Another source of hope and inspiration for cancer patients is spirituality. Patients who have a strong faith or belief system can turn to prayer, religious practices, and meditation to help them cope and gain a sense of purpose during their journey. Engaging in spiritual practices can provide a sense of inner peace, which can be beneficial in managing the stress of cancer diagnosis and treatment.

Finding hope and inspiration in oneself is another critical aspect of a cancer patient's healing journey. Learning new skills or hobbies, practicing mindfulness, or maintaining a positive outlook can help patients find meaning and purpose even amidst the struggles. Setting goals can help patients feel empowered and motivated, leading to a sense of accomplishment, which in turn fosters hope.

A cancer diagnosis can also be an opportunity for patients to reassess their life and priorities, leading to newfound inspiration. For example, a patient may decide to volunteer or start a charity to help others going through similar experiences. Doing something for others can provide a sense of purpose beyond one's individual journey, which can be incredibly empowering.

Finally, cancer patients can find hope and inspiration from their loved ones. Family and friends can provide encouragement and support by attending appointments, listening when they need someone to talk to, or helping with practical tasks. Surrounding oneself with positivity and love can help patients feel less alone in their journey, giving them strength, hope, and inspiration.

Finding hope and inspiration in the journey is crucial for cancer patients' overall well-being and recovery. Whether from support groups, spirituality, personal growth, or loved ones, sources of hope and inspiration can come in various forms to help patients stay positive, persevere through struggles, and retain a sense of purpose and meaning.

REFLECTING ON YOUR LIFE AND VALUES

Reflecting on one's life and values is an important part of the cancer survivor journey. Surviving cancer can be a life-changing experience that can lead survivors to re-evaluate their priorities and goals. Reflecting on one's life and values can help survivors gain clarity about what is truly important to them and can guide them in making important decisions about their future.

One way to reflect on one's life and values is to take time for introspection. Survivors can set aside time each day to reflect on their experiences and to think about what they've learned from their cancer journey. They can ask themselves questions such as: What did I learn from my cancer experience? What values are most important to me? What are my goals for the future?

Another way to reflect on one's life and values is to seek out support and guidance from others. Survivors can talk to friends and family members, as well as healthcare providers, counselors, or spiritual leaders. These individuals can offer guidance and support as survivors reflect on their experiences and work to align their values with their future goals.

Engaging in creative activities can also be a helpful way to reflect on one's life and values. Survivors can write in a journal, create art, or compose music as a way to process their experiences and to gain insight into their values and priorities. These activities can also serve as a form of self-expression and can help survivors to feel more empowered and in control of their lives.

Finally, survivors can reflect on their life and values by setting goals for the future. These goals can be related to personal growth, career aspirations, or relationships. By setting goals that align with their values and priorities, survivors can create a roadmap for the future that feels meaningful and fulfilling.

By reflecting on their experiences and aligning their values with their future goals, survivors can create a roadmap for the future that feels meaningful and fulfilling. Survivors should remember that their cancer journey does not define them, but rather it can serve as a source of strength and inspiration as they move forward in their lives.

CELEBRATING MILESTONES AND ACCOMPLISHMENTS

Celebrating milestones and accomplishments is an important part of the cancer survivor journey. Surviving cancer is no small feat, and every milestone and accomplishment along the way deserves to be recognized and celebrated. Celebrating milestones and accomplishments not only acknowledges the hard work and dedication it took to get there, but it also helps to boost morale and keep survivors motivated throughout their cancer journey.

There are many different milestones and accomplishments that cancer survivors can celebrate throughout their journey. Some of the most common milestones include completing treatment, reaching a specific milestone in treatment (such as the halfway point), and reaching the end of a particularly difficult treatment phase. Accomplishments can include anything from being able to eat a full meal without feeling nauseous to completing a 5K race.

One way to celebrate milestones and accomplishments is to throw a party or gather with friends and family. This can be a great way to acknowledge the hard work and dedication that went into reaching the milestone or accomplishment, as well as to share the joy with loved ones. Survivors can also choose to celebrate privately, by treating themselves to a special meal, taking a day off work, or indulging in a favorite hobby.

Another way to celebrate milestones and accomplishments is to create a scrapbook or journal. This can be a great way to document the journey and to remember all of the hard work and dedication that went into reaching each milestone and accomplishment. Survivors can include photos, mementos, and journal entries to help them remember the journey and to celebrate their successes.

Cancer survivors can also celebrate milestones and accomplishments by giving back to others. Survivors can volunteer at a cancer center or hospital, participate in a cancer fundraising event, or simply offer support and encouragement to other survivors. Giving back can be a great way to celebrate one's own journey while also helping others who are just starting their own.

Finally, survivors can celebrate milestones and accomplishments by taking time to reflect on their journey and to set new goals for the future. Survivors can use their accomplishments as motivation to keep pushing forward and to set new goals for themselves. Whether it's learning a new skill, taking a trip, or simply enjoying time with loved ones, survivors can use their milestones and accomplishments as a springboard for new opportunities and experiences.

Celebrating milestones and accomplishments is an important part of the cancer survivor journey. Surviving cancer is a major accomplishment, and survivors should take the time to acknowledge and celebrate their hard work and dedication. Whether it's throwing a party, creating a scrapbook, giving back to others, or setting new goals for the future, survivors should embrace every opportunity to celebrate their journey and to continue moving forward with strength and resilience.

MANAGING FEAR AND ANXIETY ABOUT RECURRENCE

Managing fear and anxiety about recurrence is a common challenge for cancer survivors. After completing treatment, many survivors worry about the possibility of cancer returning. This fear and anxiety can be overwhelming and can significantly impact a survivor's quality of life. However, there are strategies that survivors can use to manage their fear and anxiety and to live their lives to the fullest.

One of the most effective strategies for managing fear and anxiety about recurrence is to stay informed about one's health. Survivors can work with their healthcare team to develop a follow-up plan that includes regular check-ups and screenings. Knowing that one is taking proactive steps to monitor their health can help to alleviate some of the fear and anxiety about recurrence.

Another important strategy is to practice self-care. This can include anything from getting enough rest and exercise to eating a healthy diet and practicing stress-reduction techniques such as meditation or deep breathing. Self-care can help to reduce stress and anxiety, which can in turn improve overall well-being and quality of life.

Support from loved ones can also be incredibly helpful in managing fear and anxiety about recurrence. Survivors can reach out to friends and family members for emotional support and encouragement. They can also join support groups or connect with other survivors who have gone through similar experiences. Talking to others who understand what it's like to live with the fear of recurrence can be incredibly validating and can help to reduce feelings of isolation.

Cognitive-behavioral therapy (CBT) is another effective strategy for managing fear and anxiety about recurrence. CBT is a type of therapy that helps individuals identify and change negative thought patterns and behaviors. By challenging negative thoughts and replacing them with more positive and realistic ones, CBT can help to reduce anxiety and improve overall well-being.

Finally, survivors can also work to shift their perspective about cancer and recurrence. While it's natural to feel afraid and anxious about the possibility of cancer returning, survivors can choose to focus on the present moment and on the things that bring them joy and fulfillment. They can also focus on the positive aspects of their journey, such as the strength and resilience they've developed as a result of their experience.

Staying informed about one's health, practicing self-care, seeking support from loved ones, engaging in cognitive-behavioral therapy, and shifting one's perspective can all be effective strategies for managing fear and anxiety about recurrence. Survivors should remember that while the fear of recurrence may never completely go away, it is possible to live a fulfilling and meaningful life after cancer.

EMBRACING LIFE AFTER CANCER

Being diagnosed with cancer can be a life-altering experience. Surviving cancer, however, can be just as transformative. Embracing life after cancer is an essential part of the journey towards healing and recovery. It can be a time to reflect on what truly matters in life, to find new meaning and purpose, and to find joy and fulfillment in the present moment.

One of the most important aspects of embracing life after cancer is learning to live in the present moment. Cancer survivors often experience a range of emotions, including fear, anxiety, and uncertainty about the future. It can be easy to get caught up in worries about recurrence or the long-term effects of treatment. However, by learning to focus on the present moment, survivors can find peace and joy in the here and now. This might involve practicing mindfulness, meditation, or other relaxation techniques that help to quiet the mind and center the body.

Another key component of embracing life after cancer is finding a sense of purpose and meaning. Cancer can be a wake-up call, prompting survivors to re-evaluate their priorities and make changes in their lives. For some, this might mean pursuing a new career, volunteering for a cause that is meaningful to them, or spending more time with loved ones. For others, it might involve exploring spirituality or creative pursuits, such as art or writing. Whatever the path, finding purpose and meaning can be a powerful way to move forward and create a fulfilling life after cancer.

Physical activity can also play a vital role in embracing life after cancer. Exercise has been shown to have numerous physical and psychological benefits for cancer survivors. It can help to reduce fatigue, improve mood, and increase overall energy levels. Additionally, regular exercise can help to reduce the risk of recurrence and improve overall health and well-being. Finding an exercise routine that is enjoyable and sustainable can be an important part of creating a healthy, vibrant life after cancer.

Social support is another key ingredient in embracing life after cancer. Connecting with others who have shared similar experiences can be incredibly validating and empowering. Support groups, online forums, and other resources can provide a sense of community and a safe space for survivors to share their feelings and concerns. Additionally, spending time with friends and loved ones can provide a sense of normalcy and connection that is essential for emotional healing and recovery.

Finally, it is important for cancer survivors to prioritize self-care in their lives. This might involve making time for activities that bring joy and relaxation, such as reading, taking a bath, or getting a massage. It could also involve adopting healthy habits, such as eating a nutritious diet, getting enough sleep, and avoiding unhealthy behaviors like smoking or excessive drinking. By taking care of themselves, survivors can ensure that they have the physical, emotional, and mental resources they need to create a fulfilling life after cancer.

In conclusion, embracing life after cancer is a journey that requires patience, courage, and resilience. It is about finding new ways to live a fulfilling life, even in the face of adversity. By focusing on the present moment, finding purpose and meaning, engaging in physical activity, seeking social support, and prioritizing self-care, cancer survivors can move forward with confidence and hope for the future.

PART VI

CONCLUSION

THE JOURNEY OF HEALING: A CONTINUING PROCESS

The journey of healing for cancer survivors is a continuous process that evolves over time. It is not a one-time event that ends with the completion of treatment or the achievement of remission. Instead, healing is a lifelong process that involves physical, emotional, and spiritual well-being.

For many cancer survivors, the journey of healing begins with the diagnosis itself. It is a time of shock, fear, and uncertainty, as they come to terms with the reality of their illness. Treatment can be challenging, with its side effects and the toll it takes on the body. However, the journey of healing is about more than just physical recovery.

Emotional healing is an essential aspect of the journey of healing. Cancer survivors may experience a range of emotions, including fear, anxiety, anger, and depression. These feelings are normal and understandable, given the trauma of the cancer experience. However, it is important to find ways to process and cope with these emotions, rather than bottling them up or denying their existence. This might involve seeking therapy, joining a support group, or practicing self-care activities that promote emotional well-being.

Spiritual healing is another important aspect of the journey of healing. For some cancer survivors, cancer can be a spiritual wake-up call, prompting them to re-evaluate their beliefs and priorities. Spirituality can provide a sense of meaning and purpose, as well as a source of comfort and support during difficult times. Whether through prayer, meditation, or other spiritual practices, finding a sense of connection to something greater than oneself can be a powerful tool for healing.

The journey of healing is not a linear process. There may be setbacks, challenges, and unexpected twists and turns along the way. However, with time and patience, survivors can learn to navigate these challenges and find new ways of living a fulfilling life. Healing is not about erasing the past or forgetting the trauma of cancer. Instead, it is about finding a way to integrate the cancer experience into one's life story, and to find meaning and purpose in the face of adversity.

Ultimately, the journey of healing is a personal one, and there is no one-size-fits-all approach. Each survivor must find their own path to healing, based on their unique needs and circumstances. However, there are common themes and principles that can guide the process. These include focusing on the present moment, finding purpose and meaning, engaging in physical activity, seeking social support, prioritizing self-care, and embracing the journey of healing as a continuous process.

In conclusion, the journey of healing for cancer survivors is a complex and ongoing process that involves physical, emotional, and spiritual well-being. It is a journey that requires patience, courage, and resilience, but it is also a journey that can be transformative and empowering. By embracing the journey of healing as a continuous process, survivors can find new ways to live a fulfilling life, even in the face of adversity.

APPENDIX: ADDITIONAL RESOURCES FOR CANCER PATIENTS AND CAREGIVERS

There are many resources available to support cancer patients and their loved ones through the cancer journey. This appendix provides a list of additional resources for cancer patients and caregivers to help them find the support they need.

SUPPORT GROUPS

Cancer support groups are a valuable resource for cancer patients and their caregivers. They provide a safe space for people to share their experiences, ask questions, and receive emotional support from others who are going through similar experiences. Support groups can be in-person or online and may be specific to certain types of cancer or stages of treatment. Some popular cancer support groups include the American Cancer Society's Cancer Survivors Network, CancerCare, and the Leukemia & Lymphoma Society's Community Support.

FINANCIAL ASSISTANCE

Cancer treatment can be expensive, and many cancer patients and their families struggle with the financial burden of treatment. Fortunately, there are organizations that provide financial assistance to cancer patients and their families. The Cancer

Financial Assistance Coalition (CFAC) is a nonprofit organization that provides a database of financial resources for cancer patients. The Patient Advocate Foundation (PAF) is another nonprofit organization that provides financial assistance and advocacy services for patients with chronic, life-threatening, or debilitating illnesses. Additionally, many cancer treatment centers have financial counselors who can help patients and their families navigate the financial aspects of cancer treatment.

TRANSPORTATION ASSISTANCE

Getting to and from cancer treatment appointments can be a challenge for many patients, especially those who live far away from treatment centers or who are too sick to drive. Fortunately, there are organizations that provide transportation assistance to cancer patients. The American Cancer Society's Road to Recovery program provides free transportation to and from cancer treatment for patients who do not have a ride or are unable to drive themselves. The National Patient Travel Center is another organization that provides travel assistance to patients who need to travel for medical treatment.

NUTRITION AND EXERCISE

Eating a healthy diet and staying physically active can help cancer patients manage treatment side effects, improve their overall health, and reduce their risk of recurrence. Many cancer treatment centers have nutritionists and exercise specialists who can provide guidance and support to patients. Additionally, there are organizations that provide free or low-cost nutrition and exercise programs for cancer patients, such as the Cancer Support Community's Frankly Speaking About Cancer program and the LIVESTRONG Foundation's Livestrong at the YMCA program.

CAREGIVER SUPPORT

Caring for a loved one with cancer can be a challenging and stressful experience. Caregivers may struggle with balancing their own needs with the needs of their loved one, managing treatment side effects, and coping with the emotional toll of caregiving. Fortunately, there are resources available to support caregivers. The Family Caregiver Alliance is a nonprofit organization that provides information, education, and support to caregivers. The National Cancer Institute's Coping with Cancer as a Caregiver website provides resources and information specifically for cancer caregivers. Additionally, many cancer treatment centers have support groups or counseling services for caregivers.

ONLINE RESOURCES

The internet can be a valuable resource for cancer patients and their caregivers. There are many online resources available that provide information, support, and community for cancer patients and their loved ones. The American Cancer Society's website provides comprehensive information on cancer diagnosis, treatment, and support

Printed in Great Britain
by Amazon